The Sinus Solution

The Ultimate Guide to Getting Permanent Relief From Chronic Sinusitis

Seth H. Evans, M.D.

ISBN: 1548113336
ISBN-13: 978-1548113339

DEDICATION

To Eliza Evans, for inspiring me to show kindness,
generosity, and love to everyone without exception.

CONTENTS

ACKNOWLEDGMENTS

I would like to thank all the teachers I had through my many years of schooling and training, but especially my mentors at Virginia Commonwealth University who taught me to be a judicious surgeon.

I thank my parents, Bobby and Pam Evans, for their unwavering support for me and my dreams, and the solid foundation they provided for my life.

And finally, I thank my partner and best friend, Renee Evans, for her faith in me and her dedication to us.

1 IS IT REALLY POSSIBLE TO GET LASTING RELIEF FROM CHRONIC SINUSITIS?

The answer to that question, in my experience, is a definite yes. I've been treating sinus problems for more than seven years, and if you include my training, more than 12 years. I've seen a lot of people get great results and long lasting improvement in their chronic sinus problems.

If you're reading this book, I'm going to assume that you are a regular person, not a doctor or someone in the medical field. I see regular people like you all the time in my office, and very few realize that there are a lot of great options for treating chronic sinus problems. Too many people assume that their lives will just be an endless cycle of antibiotics and decongestants, with all-too-short interludes of feeling decent in between. Some of them know of friends or relatives who had some sort of barbaric-sounding sinus surgery years ago, and ended up with a painful recovery, a nose stuffed with gauze packing for days after the surgery, and after all that misery, no improvement in their sinuses.

I'm here to tell you today that amazing advances have been made in how we are able to treat chronic sinus infections. Just in the last 10 years, a simple and safe procedure has been developed that has transformed the way that sinus doctors can treat your sinuses. This procedure can be done easily and comfortably in 30 minutes or less in your doctor's office, not in a hospital operating room.

So, if you're one of the many people out there suffering in silence with chronic sinusitis or never-ending sinus infections, I wrote this book for you. My purpose is to let you know about the great treatments available in 2017 for what many people still consider to be unsolvable problems.

First, who am I?

My name is Dr. Seth Evans. I first decided I wanted to be a doctor when I was about 10 years old. I was always fascinated by helping people, healing people, and the intricate complexity of how our bodies work. I studied hard and ended up getting admitted to medical school. While I was in medical school, I became very interested in the specialty of ear, nose and throat medicine during my gross anatomy class.

To keep us first-year medical students more interested, our anatomy course director would bring in actual clinical doctors to talk about surgeries and other practical aspects of what we were learning. I still remember the fascination I felt the day that the ENT surgeon lectured to us and showed pictures and videos of all the amazing surgeries that he did.

That lecture in anatomy class planted the seed in my mind about ENT as my future specialty. Over the rest of medical school, I spent more time getting to know this field, and ruling out other specialties. Ultimately, I chose to apply to ENT for my residency training and made this my goal for my future career in medicine. I liked the complex anatomy of the head and neck and I wasn't very interested in poop, feet, and the other end of the body, so ENT was a great choice for me.

Why am I interested in sinus surgery in particular?

I think part of it is that I grew up playing video games, and doing sinus surgery is actually a lot like playing video games. When I perform sinus surgery, everything happens on a TV screen. I use a camera to look inside the nose and have little instruments that go inside the nose. I think the video game skillset transferred over nicely to doing sinus procedures.

I don't actually play video games anymore because I would probably spend all my time doing that instead of more important things! But, I have definitely discovered that treating sinus problems is

3

incredibly rewarding and interesting to me. And it's not always surgery either- many times I'm able to find excellent ways of treating these problems with medications, allergy therapy, or office procedures. If you're reading this book, I know I can help you with your sinus problems too.

This book is for people with chronic sinusitis or recurrent sinus infections who want to get long-lasting relief from their never-ending sinus issues. It is not for people who only get one sinus infection a year or maybe two infections a year. The people I am interested in reaching through this book are those who are getting at least 3 sinus infections every year or having chronic sinus symptoms that are not getting better for months or years on end. If you are one of those people, and you think that you will never get better, I know I have some options to help you get relief.

I would like now to tell a brief story about something that happened in the fall of 2012 which changed my way of treating people who have chronic sinusitis. This was shortly after I started my practice in Texas. I had a teenage girl come into my office, complaining of never ending sinus problems. For years and years, she had been congested all the time, with lots of pressure in her face. She was blowing lot of thick stuff out of her nose, and she was just miserable. In the past, I would have offered sinus surgery for her, but I had learned about a relatively new sinus procedure that had been out for only a few years.

By 2012, this procedure had been developed and improved to the point where it had become much more widespread and common. The procedure is called balloon sinuplasty. I decided to offer it for my young patient and see how well it worked. I took her to the operating room and did the procedure under anesthesia. Since then, I've done more than 150 of these procedures in my office, not in the operating room.

So what is balloon sinuplasty?

We'll talk much more about balloon sinuplasty later in the book, but in short this procedure involves permanently widening the narrow sinus openings inside your nose by inflating a small balloon to stretch them open.

My first balloon procedure went smoothly, and then I saw my young patient back a couple weeks later in the office. I can still picture it in my mind: she just came in with a huge smile on her face and she already was feeling much better, breathing better, and her whole life was starting to transform. Over the next couple of months, I continued to see this patient in follow-up and it was the same story each time. She was so happy and glad she had the balloon procedure. It was not a difficult recovery for her and she was really excited and feeling great.

Since then, I've developed a lot more experience with this procedure and I'm convinced it is the right option for many people like you who are sick and tired of never-ending sinus infections and congestion.

The purpose of this book is to give you an understanding of what is chronic sinusitis, what are the various options for treating it, and then we're going to focus on the balloon sinuplasty procedure in detail.

2 WHAT IS SINUSITIS?

Before we start talking about how to treat sinusitis, we need to understand what it is! There is a lot of confusion out there about whether symptoms like headache or congestion are caused by a sinus infection or by something else. Even many doctors get confused by this.

In this chapter, you will learn how ENT doctors like myself diagnose sinusitis.

Does sinusitis equal a sinus infection?

Not necessarily. The word sinusitis is composed of "sinus" and "itis" which means inflammation. So "sinusitis" means inflammation of the sinuses. Infection is a possible cause of inflammation but many other things can cause inflammation, most commonly allergies. However, the term sinusitis and sinus infection are frequently used interchangeably. We'll use both of those terms throughout the rest of this book, but it is important for you to understand that not all sinusitis is caused by infection.

What are the sinuses?

The sinuses are hollow spaces inside of your head. They are sometimes called the paranasal sinuses ("para" means around, so paranasal means around the nasal cavity). All the sinuses open up into the inside of your nose and normally drain mucus out that way. All the lining inside your nose and sinuses produces mucus all the time. In a normal situation, this mucus drains into your nose and you never notice it.

You have a total of four paranasal sinuses on each side. There's the maxillary sinuses, which are in your cheeks under your eyes. The frontal sinuses, which are in your forehead. The sphenoid sinuses, which are in the very back of the nose. And finally the ethmoid sinuses, which are in between the eyes.

Paranasal sinuses

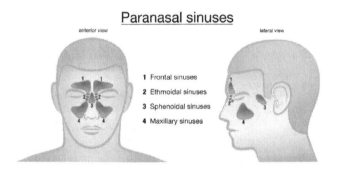

anterior view   lateral view

1 Frontal sinuses
2 Ethmoidal sinuses
3 Sphenoidal sinuses
4 Maxillary sinuses

Three of those four sinuses, the maxillary, the frontal and the sphenoid are similar in that they're one big open space with one opening out into the inside of the nose. The ethmoid sinuses are different. They're more like small little connected pockets like a honeycomb. Those are the four sets of sinuses- you have one set of each of them on each side of your face.

Why do we have sinuses?

I don't think anybody knows for sure, but there are a few theories of why we have sinuses. The first hypothesis is that the sinuses make our heads lighter. The idea is that humans evolved to have large heavy brains so that we can be more intelligent, and without having some sort of air filled spaces in our heads, our heads would become too heavy to hold up.

Another theory is that the sinuses act as a crumple zone, so if you get hit in the face, your face will crunch and crumble before you sustain damage to your brain, eyeballs, or other more important structures. This is similar to how your car was made. If you ran head-on into a brick wall at 60 miles per hour, the front of your car is designed to crumple up and absorb the force of impact, so less of that force is transferred to you and anyone riding with you.

Finally, there's the idea that the sinuses help provide resonance to our voices. When we speak, the sound of our voice echoes through the air filled spaces in our throats, mouths, and nasal cavity. Having that extra air-filled space can help make our voices louder and more resonant.

Ultimately, no one really knows why we have sinuses, but these are the most common theories that are out there.

What happens when I get sinusitis?

Again, sinusitis means inflammation of the sinuses. What does the term inflammation mean? The official definition from the dictionary is "a localized physical condition in which part of the body becomes reddened, swollen, hot, and often painful, commonly as a reaction to injury or infection."

This inflammation in the sinuses can happen for a few reasons. Very commonly, it's because the openings out of the sinuses become blocked. This can be caused by swelling from allergies or from a viral infection (a cold or the flu), but when those openings become blocked, the sinus then builds up with pressure because it cannot drain. It can collect thick and infected mucus and you'll start feeling pressure and congestion in that area. On x-rays or CT scans, I typically will see thickening of the lining inside the sinus and potentially see trapped mucus inside the sinuses.

What are the main symptoms of sinusitis?

There are four main symptoms of sinusitis. The first of these is congestion or obstruction in the nose. This means that you feel stuffy and you have a hard time breathing or passing air through your nose. The second symptom is pressure, usually above and below the eyes or between the eyes. People will sometimes call this sinus headache or sinus pressure. The third symptom is thick drainage from your nose. Most commonly this is discolored (green, yellow, or brown). Sometimes, you'll have more drainage dripping into the back of your throat than coming out the front of your nose. Finally, the fourth major symptom is smell disturbance. This can be a diminished sense of smell or a complete loss of smell.

As a quick reference, the four major symptoms of sinusitis are:

1. Nasal congestion
2. Pressure in the face
3. Thick nasal drainage
4. Diminished sense of smell

What are the minor symptoms of sinusitis?

Not all people will have these symptoms, but they do happen sometimes. These include cough, ear pain or pressure, tooth pain, fever, general fatigue/tiredness, and headaches inside the head or in the top of the head. Without any or most of the four major symptoms discussed above, it's less likely that you truly have sinusitis or a sinus infection. Very commonly, I see people who believe they have sinus problems and then they start talking about symptoms in their throats or their ears or feeling dizzy or lots of other things that don't really have anything to do with their sinuses.

The reason that we're going over all this information is that you can understand what is actually sinusitis and what isn't. Most people would not want to be treated for sinusitis when they don't really have it, especially if that treatment is a procedure or surgery.

Do I have to have all of the four major symptoms to be diagnosed with sinusitis?

You do not. It's just a good rule of thumb. Normally, I would expect most people to have at least three out of those four to feel confident in the diagnosis, though sometimes it's only two (in these cases, the diagnosis can be confirmed in other ways, such as looking inside the nose or looking at a CT scan).

If it's only 1 or zero of the main symptoms, you probably have something other than sinusitis that is causing your problem. There are more examinations and tests that we can do but a large part of diagnosing sinusitis is your story and the symptoms you are having.

What's the difference between acute and chronic sinusitis?

Acute sinusitis is what most people typically call a sinus infection. It is defined as having the symptoms of sinusitis for less than four weeks. Most of the time, you can treat this with medications like antibiotics and decongestants and it gets better. Chronic sinusitis is defined as having sinusitis symptoms that last more than 12 weeks.. In between those two extremes, we have what's called subacute sinusitis, which is defined as having symptoms between four and 12 weeks.

As a quick reference:

- Acute Sinusitis = Symptoms last for <4 weeks
- Subacute Sinusitis = Symptoms last between 4-12 weeks
- Chronic Sinusitis = Symptoms last longer than 12 weeks

What is recurrent acute sinusitis?

Recurrent acute sinusitis, by the textbook, means having four or more episodes of acute sinusitis per year. Some doctors, including myself, will consider it if you have three or more sinus infections per year.

Why do we have this as a diagnosis? Basically, the point of recurrent acute sinusitis is to have a threshold of how many sinus infections you should get each year before you should consider having surgery to treat them. In the past, when more invasive forms of surgery were required, you probably should be getting 4 or more sinus infections per year before considering surgery. Now that less invasive and safer office procedures are available, I think it makes sense to drop that to 3 infections per year.

What are nasal polyps?

Nasal polyps are sometimes seen in people who have chronic sinusitis. These are benign growths within the nose. Although they are masses inside the nose, polyps are not a type of cancer and they have no risk of turning into cancer. Polyps are overgrowths of the lining inside the nose and sinuses. When I look in the nose of a patient with nasal polyps, I see large gelatinous pale blobs of tissue. These blobs of tissue can then block the sinus openings or even block your breathing completely if they get large enough.

What is the difference between nasal allergy symptoms and sinusitis?

Allergy symptoms are different from typical sinusitis symptoms. Both of these problems have some overlap, so it is easy for people to get confused, but the main differences are as follows. With allergies, typically you'll see clear, watery drainage instead of the thicker drainage seen in sinusitis. You'll also experience more itching and sneezing in the nose rather than pressure and discomfort. Patients with bad allergies often complain of itchy and watery eyes as well.

Usually, people don't really feel sick when they have allergies. They may be tired because they are up all night blowing their noses and sneezing, but they feel okay other than their nose being stuffy or blowing their nose a lot.

What if I have migraine headaches?

Migraines are often confused with sinusitis, even by many doctors. People who complain about "sinus headaches" are much more commonly suffering from migraines than from sinusitis. The classic migraine symptoms of pounding headache, nausea, and light sensitivity do not always happen in all migraine headaches. Frequently, they can occur as facial pressure similar to sinusitis.

Migraines can also sometimes cause nasal congestion. But normally migraines do not cause the thick discolored drainage or loss of smell seen in sinusitis. It is also important to realize that people can have migraines AND sinusitis, and just because you might have migraines, it does not mean you should never have treatment for sinusitis. I see many ENT doctors that get confused about this point, and attribute all a patient's symptoms to their migraines, even if it is clear that there is sinusitis as well.

What are the three underlying causes of chronic sinusitis?

Number one is structural problems. These problems would include narrow sinus openings or other structural issues that cause blockage and drainage issues. If you imagine the sinus openings like plumbing pipes in your house, then we are talking about pipes that are too narrow and get clogged easily.

The second underlying cause of sinusitis is

inflammation or swelling of the tissues in the nose. This inflammation could be due to underlying allergy, infection, or less common problems such as certain autoimmune disorders. Finally, the third cause is true bacterial infection. This is particularly the case in chronic sinusitis patients who are colonized with an antibiotic-resistant strain of bacteria.

Not everyone has to have all three of these causes all the time. In fact, I would say that bacterial infection is probably the least common of the three. More often, I see that major structural problems (narrow pipes) and underlying inflammation and swelling due to allergy are the main issues.

So, you have now gained a lot of knowledge about sinusitis, more than many doctors! If you use the things you have learned, you should be starting to understand if you truly have chronic or recurrent sinusitis. With this knowledge, we will move on in the next chapter to learn how to treat these problems.

3 WHAT NON-SURGICAL OPTIONS CAN I USE FOR CHRONIC SINUS PROBLEMS?

Before we start rushing into a discussion of procedures or surgeries, let's talk about the many medicines and non-surgical options that are available to treat and prevent sinusitis. These treatments tend to work best for people with occasional sinus infections and other mild issues. Let's get started:

Are there any herbal or nutritional supplements that are effective?

Unfortunately, there's really no supplements that have been shown to relieve sinusitis. I've seen different blog posts and other questionable information online that claim that apple cider vinegar or cayenne pepper supplements can treat or cure sinusitis. I actually researched both of those nutritional supplements on PubMed.com, which is a very complete listing of published medical research and I found zero results for any studies that examined the effects of apple cider vinegar or cayenne pepper on sinusitis.

So, unfortunately, there's no evidence at all that these supplements really treat chronic sinus problems. I don't think they would necessarily hurt you but they're probably not going to help.

What allergy medicines are helpful?

There are a number of different allergy medicines, most of which are now sold over the counter. Probably the most helpful allergy medication for most people is a nasal steroid spray. These include over the counter medicines like Flonase or Nasacort. There are a number of prescription versions too, including Nasonex, Omnaris, and many others. In my opinion, they are all interchangeable. Steroids trigger a strong anti-inflammatory response in our bodies.

Nasal steroid sprays are meant to be used consistently every day to prevent congestion and allergic inflammation in the nose. They are less effective if you only use them sporadically to treat symptoms after the fact. If you're going to use Flonase or another steroid spray, I recommend placing the bottle by your toothbrush so it will remind you to use it every day.

Other helpful medicines include antihistamine medicines like Claritin, Zyrtec, Allegra, or Benadryl.

Antihistamines block a chemical called histamine that triggers congestion, runny nose, and itching. This can help relieve allergic inflammation and sometimes help improve symptoms of sinusitis.

Decongestants like Sudafed or Afrin spray can be helpful as well to open the nose and allow better drainage. You should be careful with decongestants, though. Oral decongestants like sudafed can make your blood pressure go up, which can be dangerous if you already have high blood pressure. Decongestant nasal sprays like Afrin work really well if you only use them for 3-5 days, but can cause serious problems if you use them longer than 1 week straight.

A stronger prescription medicine sometimes for allergies would be steroid pills that people take by mouth or a steroid injection given at your doctor's office. Oral or injectable steroids should be used with some caution, though, because they can have serious side effects, especially if used too often or for too long at a time (more than 2 weeks in a row).

Tell me about nasal saline irrigations.

Saline irrigations (also known as sinus rinses) are basically flushing out the inside of your nose with a dilute salt water solution. There are a number of different over the counter devices for this, including the Neti Pot, which is like a small water pot that is poured into the nose while you lean over the sink. There's also different squeeze bottles that you can use to flush the saline solution through your nose.

The idea behind saline irrigations is that they can flush out all the different things (pollen, dust, etc) you're allergic to and also clear out infected mucus from the nose. A lot of people love rinsing their nose and feel a lot better afterward. Saline irrigations can be very helpful and are a good maintenance medication to prevent allergy and sinus symptoms.

What antibiotics are used to treat sinusitis?

The choice of antibiotics differs somewhat depending on whether you have acute or chronic sinusitis. Usually for acute sinusitis, Amoxicillin or Doxycycline can be effective. Some doctors will use Zithromax, also known as a Z-pack, but I've found it's less likely to be effective. For chronic sinusitis, we usually will prescribe either Augmentin or Levaquin for a longer period of time to try and treat this.

What would I take if I had a penicillin allergy?

For someone with a Penicillin allergy, Levaquin would be a good option for a chronic sinusitis and for acute sinusitis, Doxycycline or Bactrim could be used.

Is sinusitis always helped by antibiotics?

Not necessarily. Antibiotics will treat a bacterial infection but not all sinusitis is actually caused by bacterial infections. Sometimes, it's a viral infection and sometimes it's just due to allergies or structural problems. In those cases, I would not expect antibiotics to be helpful. And don't forget, even if the antibiotics work, the sinusitis can always come back in the future.

What are side effects of the medications? What are the downsides?

For any medication, there's going to always be side effects and adverse reactions. It's a common saying in medicine that "all drugs are poison, it just depends on the dose." For antibiotics in particular, you can have allergic reactions to them and they frequently cause stomach upset, diarrhea or other gastrointestinal issues. Antibiotics for a lot of women also cause vaginal yeast infections, which can be very annoying.

A serious problem with antibiotics that is starting to get a lot more awareness is that antibiotics can disrupt the balance of healthy bacteria in your intestines. This can potentially lead to chronic digestive problems and at worst, can allow overgrowth of toxic bacteria called Clostridium Difficile within the intestines. It is definitely something to think about before taking antibiotics-they are not benign drugs!

For allergy medicines, people can get excessive dryness inside the nose or nosebleeds. The problem with all medications is that after you stop taking them, they'll stop working.

Is allergy testing and treatment a good idea?

Yes, allergy testing and individualized treatment like allergy shots can be very effective. For sinusitis in particular, allergy shots or other allergy treatment can help by limiting or eliminating inflammation and swelling inside the nose and sinuses that is caused by allergy. The problem with allergy therapy is that it's a slow fix for the problem.

After you are tested for allergies and start allergy shots, or other allergy treatment like sublingual allergy drops, it can take up to one year to even see if it works much less get any benefit from it. But it is effective in a lot of people. It just takes a long time to see if it will be effective.

What's the downside of medical management or allergy treatment?

I think ultimately the downside of any medical treatment is that you have to keep taking the medication either forever or for many years or otherwise it will stop working and you'll be back in the same boat again. Medical treatment can be very helpful at relieving symptoms, but it is not a permanent fix.

If we are looking for a permanent treatment, we have to start looking at fixing the structure inside of the nose. If your clogged sinuses can be opened, you now have an opportunity for long-lasting relief from your chronic sinusitis. We will learn about the various procedures and surgery available for chronic sinus problems in the next chapter.

4 WHAT SURGERIES AND PROCEDURES ARE AVAILABLE FOR CHRONIC SINUS PROBLEMS?

In this chapter, you'll learn about the current procedures and surgeries that are available for patients with chronic sinus problems. We'll start off with a brief history lesson of where sinus surgery has come from (it's not pretty!) and then move on to the much improved options for treatment today.

Isn't sinus surgery risky and painful?

In the past, yes. Fortunately, it's becoming much less risky and less painful with time. Usually these days we are able to avoid any packing in the nose and frequently avoid even going to the operating room or needing general anesthesia. Sinus surgery is definitely becoming safer and more user-friendly as technology advances.

Tell me about sinus surgery before the 1980's.

In the old days, sinus surgery was quite crude and barbaric compared to what we are able to do today. These days we would call those old forms of sinus surgery non-functional. What do I mean by the term "functional?" Let me explain. The idea to understand is that our sinuses have one opening that drains out into the nose. The lining inside the sinuses has microscopic structures called cilia which push all the mucus in the sinus toward that natural opening.

A "functional" procedure would try to unblock these natural openings into the sinuses to restore their normal function. In the old days, there was no good way to get access to those openings because fiberoptic endoscopes had not been invented yet. So surgeons would just basically punch a hole into the sinuses whichever way they could.

If you imagine one of your sinuses as a bathtub with a clogged drain, then these old forms of sinus surgery would be like blowing a hole into the side of the bathtub to fix the problem. It does help somewhat to drain the backed up water out of the bathtub, but it is not really the best way to treat it.

What is the problem with these old types of sinus surgery?

The problem with these older sinus procedures is that the tiny cilia in the lining of the sinuses want to funnel all of the mucus towards the natural opening. When surgeons created a new opening, frequently the mucus would just circulate out the natural opening back through the new opening and that would cause more problems and more severe infections that could not be treated easily.

In addition, in some of these old procedures, it is necessary that large incisions be made under the lip or up above the hairline in the scalp to get access to the sinuses and then holes would be drilled through the bone into the sinuses. These surgeries were frequently dangerous and didn't work very well because as we have said already, they were non-functional.

Is anyone still doing any of the older sinus surgeries?

These procedures and surgical approaches still have their place in modern medicine. However, they are typically used now for removal of tumors, repair after facial trauma, or other unusual reasons. The generations of surgeons who trained in these methods for treatment of sinusitis have now almost completely retired. Fortunately, we have developed new and better ways to treat chronic sinusitis, as you will now learn about.

What is FESS?

FESS stands for functional endoscopic sinus surgery. This was a technique developed in the early 1980's, and it was a great improvement over what was available before. The main word is "functional" and the big advancement was that surgeons were actually starting to address where the problem was, which was the natural opening into the sinuses.

Endoscopic means that we surgeons use a telescope to look inside the nose, so no external skin incisions are necessary anymore. In a nutshell, FESS involves looking into the nose with the scope and widening the natural openings into the sinuses by cutting and removing tissue and bone. There are a number of specialized instruments available to help me to do this job.

FESS was the main method of sinus surgery that I learned during my residency training from 2005-2010. It is still a great procedure for many patients with chronic sinusitis and endoscopic sinus surgery is one of my favorite types of surgery to perform. If you remember my video game analogy from the first chapter, FESS is the procedure I was talking about.

How was FESS received in the 1980's?

When this procedure was introduced, it was quite controversial. I think doctors, as a whole, tend to be conservative and don't like to change. At that point in time, every ENT doctor in the world had trained to do the old types of surgery, and then this newfangled endoscopic procedure was introduced onto the scene and there was a lot of controversy about it. Older doctors were not used to working with endoscopes, and they did not have the skillset necessary to effectively and safely perform FESS.

Initially, I think that FESS was a fairly dangerous procedure because a lot of these older doctors would just take a weekend course and then start doing these procedures and there are some serious complications if surgeons don't know what they are doing. We will discuss the potential complications of FESS later, but fortunately they are not common in experienced hands.

Is FESS effective?

Absolutely, and it is a great advance over the older forms of sinus surgery. These days, FESS is still an excellent option for chronic sinusitis, especially for people who have large nasal polyps or who have had previous sinus surgery.

If we go back to our bathtub analogy from above, then FESS is like cutting a hole in the bottom of the bathtub where the drain is. It makes a lot more sense than blasting a hole in the side of the tub, but it is still somewhat crude.

What are the risks of FESS?

For any procedure in the nose, there's always a risk of a bad nosebleed afterwards, or scarring inside the nose. Specifically for endoscopic sinus surgery, there is a risk of either cerebrospinal fluid leak from around the brain or injury to the eye socket and the eyeball. The reason for this is that the sidewall of the nasal cavity is the inside wall of the eye socket and the roof of the nasal cavity is the floor under the brain. These are thin areas of bone, and can easily be injured, especially in inexperienced hands. For patients having FESS by a well-trained surgeon with good sinus surgical experience, the risk of either of these complications is about 1%.

What is balloon sinuplasty?

Balloon sinuplasty is a procedure introduced in 2004. It is really doing the same thing as FESS, but there's no removal or cutting of tissue. Instead of cutting out tissue and bone to widen the sinus openings, in balloon sinuplasty the sinus openings are stretched open with a balloon that is placed into the sinus opening and inflated there.

With this balloon procedure, it is possible to open up the maxillary, frontal, and sphenoid sinuses, but not the ethmoid sinuses. The reason, if you remember, is that the ethmoid sinuses are a collection of small pockets and are not one large sinus with one opening.

However, even though we can not directly treat the ethmoid sinuses, about 87% of the time, they get better if the other sinuses are opened with the balloon. Since I have started doing balloon sinuplasty procedures, I find that I am doing a lot fewer FESS procedures, especially ethmoid sinus procedures, than in the past.

Let's return to the clogged bathtub analogy one more time. If we are trying to drain our clogged bathtub, then the old pre-1980 forms of sinus surgery are like blasting a hole in the side of the bathtub, and FESS is like cutting a hole where the clogged drain is located. In contrast, balloon sinuplasty is like unclogging the existing drain and stretching it wider without cutting anything out. You don't have to be a doctor to understand that this makes good sense.

Is balloon sinuplasty effective?

Yes. There have been more and more research studies that show positive outcomes over the past 10 years. Overall, we have seen excellent results for chronic sinusitis and recurrent acute sinusitis with this procedure. One particular study saw that 95% of patients who had balloon sinuplasty still had relief over nine months after the procedures. There are also some research studies with data that covers five or more years after the procedure. This data continues to show excellent results and relief from chronic sinus symptoms.

I don't want to spend a lot of time diving into the weeds of medical research studies, but I will list references for a number of published studies in the resources section at the end of this book. If you are interested in this information, that will be a good place to start. You can also do a literature search of your own at PubMed.com.

My personal experience with this procedure corroborates these great results. Some of the happiest patients I see in my practice are people who have had balloon sinuplasty and are coming back feeling better.

What are the benefits of balloon sinuplasty versus FESS?

The first major benefit is that balloon sinuplasty

is literally 100 times safer in terms of significant or serious complications. The risk of cerebrospinal fluid leak or injury to the eye socket are about 1% for FESS, but they're less than 1 in 10,000 for balloon sinuplasty. There are many studies containing thousands of patients where there were zero serious complications. With the particular device I use to perform balloon sinuplasty (the Acclarent Spin device), it is almost inconceivable that either CSF leak or injury to the eye socket could occur. Balloon sinuplasty is extremely safe.

The next benefit versus FESS is that balloon sinuplasty can be done in the office rather than in an operating room or hospital. You don't need to get general anesthesia, fast overnight, or spend all day at the hospital for this short procedure. I am usually able to get patients in and out of the office in under an hour for their balloon sinuplasty procedures, with the actual procedure taking around 15 minutes most of the time. Finally, the recovery after having the balloon procedure is noticeably easier and less painful than after having FESS.

What are the risks of balloon sinuplasty versus FESS?

For any sinus procedure, there are always risks of cerebrospinal fluid leak or injury to the eye socket. Again, the risk with balloon sinuplasty is about one in 10,000 versus one in 100 for FESS. I have not seen either of these complications in over 200 balloon sinuplasties I have performed (this includes procedures in the office and in the operating room).

I think that even if one of these somehow happened in a balloon sinuplasty procedure, the only way it could happen would be a small crack in the bone, not a large injury. The Acclarent Spin device I use in the balloon sinuplasty procedure has a guide wire that I gently advance to find the sinus opening and there's literally no way you can push a guide wire where it shouldn't go. Thus, the risk of a serious injury like the ones described above is very, very low.

Is balloon sinuplasty controversial?

Balloon sinuplasty is still somewhat controversial, and a lot of the same arguments that occurred during the transition from the old pre-1980 forms of sinus surgery to FESS are echoing again now in the transition from FESS to using the balloon. The consensus among the ENT community is slowly shifting in favor of the balloon.

This shift is for two main reasons: first, each year more and more research studies are published that confirm the effectiveness and safety of this procedure. And second, more and more surgeons are performing balloon sinuplasty and getting experience with it. I like to say that the only surgeon who thinks balloon sinuplasty doesn't work is the surgeon who never does it. I've performed over 200 of these procedures as of this writing, and it is blindingly obvious to me that balloon sinuplasty works and it helps people.

But you may see differing opinions online or if

you end up seeing another ENT doctor. My advice to you if you find yourself in front of a doctor who disparages balloon sinuplasty would be to ask him or her how many of these procedures they have personally done. If the answer is "none" or "I did one once 2 years ago and it didn't work" or something similar, I would advise you to consider looking for a second opinion. Ultimately, you have to review all the sides of the debate for yourself and decide what is best for you.

In conclusion, you have now learned about the history of sinus surgery from the old invasive methods through to the current technologies we have available like the balloon sinuplasty procedure. Now, I will give you my advice on how to decide between all the various treatment options.

5 HOW DO I DECIDE WHAT TREATMENT OR PROCEDURE IS RIGHT FOR ME?

In this chapter, I will tell you how I think about chronic sinusitis and other persistent sinus problems. I'll give you the algorithms and thought processes I use to make decisions on what to recommend for different patients who come to me for treatment of their sinus issues.

What do you recommend for people who get acute sinusitis two times a year or fewer?

These are people who just get an occasional sinus infection. Almost everyone gets a sinus infection at some point in their lives. You do not need surgery or procedure if you are one of these people. Most likely if you have taken the time to get this far in the book, your sinus problems are more severe. For those with only occasional sinus infections, I typically would prescribe antibiotics, decongestants and possibly steroids, but they definitely do not need any surgery or procedure.

What do you recommend for recurrent acute sinusitis?

If you remember from Chapter 2, these are people who get three or more sinus infections every year. They usually tell me story of getting prescribed antibiotics or other treatment and each sinus infection clears up, but within a few weeks or months, it is back again like a bad horror movie monster.

If you are one of these recurrent sinusitis patients, balloon sinuplasty works extremely well. After you have balloon sinuplasty, there is no guarantee you will never have another sinus infection again. But I've taken dozens of patients from having more than 3 infections per year down to one or none each year. Not only do the sinus infections usually become much less frequent, they are typically a lot easier to treat and clear out more quickly when they do occur.

What do you recommend for chronic sinusitis?

As a reminder, chronic sinusitis refers to patients who have 12 or more weeks of sinusitis symptoms. They're just not getting better. Normally, by the time these patients get in to see me, an ENT specialist, they have already been on one or more antibiotics, allergy medications, and/or steroids and have not had any real improvement.

I also believe the balloon sinuplasty is the first line treatment for most patients with chronic sinusitis, assuming that medications have not been helpful.

As we will discuss later in this chapter, FESS still remains the best option for some patients with chronic sinusitis. Examples of patients for whom I would normally recommend FESS are people with large nasal polyps filling the nose, or people who have already had FESS in the past who are now having recurrent sinus problems.

What exams and tests are needed as part of a complete sinus evaluation?

Every patient should always have a good history taken by their doctor and a sinus-focused physical exam. In my practice, I will start by talking to you and listen to the story of your sinus problems, usually asking directed questions to narrow down the diagnosis. Then I will exam your ears, nose, mouth, and neck. During the typical physical exam for a new sinus patient, I will take a detailed look in the front of your nose and press on your face over your maxillary and frontal sinuses to assess for pain and discomfort that might indicate sinusitis in these areas.

Additionally, for patients with chronic sinus problems, I will use a fiberoptic endoscope to look inside of the nose. This is a camera shaped like a thin metal straw. The endoscope slides gently inside of the nose. When I am looking inside your nose with it, it feels a little weird and uncomfortable but isn't painful. The endoscope allows me to see the general appearance of the nasal cavity and examine the areas where the sinuses are draining out that are not visible just looking in the front. I can also look for other structural problems like bone spurs off the nasal septum, scarring, or nasal polyps.

Finally, I recommend that you have a CT scan of your sinuses. CT stands for computed tomography. This is basically a fancy x-ray machine that allows me to see inside of your sinuses and note if any mucus is trapped there or if there are other signs of inflammation like thickened lining in the sinuses. The CT also shows me the dimensions of your actual sinus openings- frequently we can see exactly where those openings are blocked and narrowed. A CT scan is just like an x-ray, so it is not invasive or painful in any way. There is no need for IV contrast like there is for CT scans of some other parts of the body.

What do you recommend for patients with nasal polyps?

For nasal polyps, I can usually see them immediately by looking in the nose. This may require the nasal endoscope, but if polyps are large enough, they can be seen just by looking in the front of the nose. Every patient with a mass inside the nose needs a CT scan to make sure that the mass is actually a nasal polyp and is not a part of the brain that is extending down into the nose. Yes this happens! It is called a meningocele and (fortunately) it is pretty rare.

But I never want to go in and cut anything that looks like a polyp out of the nose until I know for sure from the CT scan that it is not part of the brain. Once I am sure that the polyp really is a polyp, patients will need to go to the operating room for a FESS surgery to remove the polyps and to open the blocked sinuses.

What about a deviated septum?

The septum is the wall down the middle of the inside of your nose. In some people, this wall is crooked and blocks one side of the nose or the other (sometimes it twists and turns so much that it blocks both sides!).

There is a surgery called septoplasty that I perform to straighten a deviated septum. Some patients with chronic sinusitis will also have a deviated septum (which may or may not be a contributing cause of their sinusitis). If the deviated septum is causing significant blockage of airflow on one side of the nose, it should be fixed. Also, if it is blocking access to the sinus openings so that I'm not able to perform any sinus procedure, it would need to be straightened primarily to allow me access to address the sinus openings.

I am fairly conservative in recommending septoplasty. No one has a perfectly straight septum, and just because your septum is mildly deviated does not mean it needs to be fixed. I can sometimes perform septoplasty in the office if the deviated area is limited to the front half of the nasal cavity. If the deviation of the septum is more severe or located farther back in the nose, I would need to go to the operating room to fix it.

What about the turbinates?

The turbinates are structures inside the nose that run along the floor of the nasal cavity from the front of the nose near the nostrils back to where the nose joins into the top of the throat. These structures are mostly composed of tissue that can expand and contract, depending on blood flow.

In people with chronic sinus problems and allergies, the turbinates tend to be swollen and expanded all the time. This causes these people to feel congested and stuffy most or all of the time. They will frequently complain of congestion that moves back and forth between the two sides of their nose every few hours.

Frequently, if patients are having balloon sinuplasty, I also recommend to shrink the turbinates at the same time. Doing this helps patients to breathe better and only takes about one or two minutes to do during the procedure. Turbinate reduction is done with a thin probe that is advanced inside the swollen tissue. Once it is placed in the right spot, the probe delivers an electric current that "cooks" the inside of the tissue of the turbinate. Over the next few weeks, the turbinate gradually shrinks down, allowing for better airflow through the nose.

Do you ever recommend allergy testing?

Yes, I do frequently. I think treating chronic

sinusitis can be looked at from two directions. One is the structural aspect, in which procedures like balloon sinuplasty or FESS are used to open the sinuses. Basically, we are widening the pipes.

The other direction is by treating allergies and other underlying inflammation. By doing this, there will be less congestion and swelling, and therefore the sinus openings are less likely to become blocked. I think both of these ways of treatment are helpful for most patients. However, I typically recommend having a procedure such as balloon sinuplasty first and then getting allergy testing later if needed.

Why is balloon sinuplasty the best option in most cases?

I think it's the best option for several reasons. First, it's very effective. The medical research supports doing balloon sinuplasty and my experience of over 200 of these procedures is also in agreement with this conclusion. It works.

Secondly, it provides quick results. Usually you will start to feel better within a week of having the procedure. If you opt for allergy shots or sublingual allergy drops, it might take up to a year for you to start feeling better.

Third, balloon sinuplasty is very low risk when compared to FESS or other forms of surgery. We already discussed this, but as a reminder, balloon sinuplasty is literally 100 times safer than FESS in terms of severe complications like eye injury or leak of cerebrospinal fluid.

Finally, balloon sinuplasty does not burn any bridges. By this, I mean that every other treatment is still available after you have had a balloon sinuplasty. If it doesn't work, all the other options are still there for you. You can still have FESS, you can still get allergy shots, and you can still take any medications available.

When would you recommend FESS over balloon sinuplasty?

I will always recommend FESS for patients with large nasal polyps that fill the nose. There is really only one good option for people with this problem, and that is to go in and cut out the polyps. A balloon is not going to remove polyps, unfortunately. For patients with chronic sinusitis and one or two small polyps, I am usually able to remove them and still perform balloon sinuplasty safely and effectively.

Patients that have had previous sinus surgery also usually need to have FESS. Usually these patients will already have large openings into the sinuses from their previous surgery and their issue is scarring or limited areas of blockage. The balloon is usually not a good option for these patients. Sometimes it still can be used, though. An example would be a patient who previously had FESS to open their maxillary sinuses but now has developed chronic frontal and sphenoid sinusitis.

So, now we have covered the typical treatments

that I recommend for patients with different types of sinus problems. For most people, balloon sinuplasty is the best first-line treatment in my opinion.

Now, we will move on to describe the typical experience of a patient in my practice who seeks me out for treatment of chronic sinusitis, starting with their first visit in the office through their balloon sinuplasty procedure and beyond.

6 WHAT HAPPENS AFTER I MAKE AN APPOINTMENT FOR MY SINUS PROBLEMS?

To start out, this is just how I do it in my practice. Every doctor is going to do things their own way, but I will tell you what your experience would be like in my practice from the time you decide to make an appointment with me through your balloon sinuplasty procedure and after the procedure.

What happens before my first office visit?

Before you come in for your appointment, my office staff will contact your health insurance and make sure we are in network with your plan. If a referral from your primary care doctor is needed, we can help contact his or her office to get the referral paperwork sent over. My staff does their best to find out how much the visit will cost out of pocket for you and we'll find out if there's any additional charge for you for nasal endoscopy or CT scans during your visit.

Sometimes the cost of these diagnostic procedures and tests is included with your office visit, but sometimes it is in addition and will be applied toward your annual deductible. It all depends on your particular insurance plan, and we try to find out that information before you come in.

Your responsibility is to complete our new patient paperwork, which is available on my practice's website at texanent.com. This paperwork includes a survey of sinus symptoms, called the Sino-Nasal Outcome Test (SNOT-20 survey). You can either download and print these papers and fill out at home or you can fill them out in the waiting room before your appointment. If you decide to fill them out in the waiting room, I request that you arrive about 15 minutes before your appointment time.

What happens when I arrive for my first appointment?

You'll come into the office and check in with my receptionist. After you hand in your completed new patient paperwork, one of my nurses will call you back to the exam room and get some basic information about why you are coming into the office today. She will take your blood pressure and other vital signs, and finally will spray a decongestant and numbing solution into your nose to help me examine it.

What history does Dr. Evans ask about?

After listening to your story in your own words, I will clarify any details about how long you've been having your sinus and nasal problems and ask you specific questions about what symptoms you are having. I focus on the major symptoms of sinusitis that we discussed earlier in chapter 2.

I will ask you about any previous medical treatments for sinusitis, including antibiotics, steroids, or allergy treatments. I will also ask about any previous surgeries you've had on your nose or your sinuses and any previous testing, including allergy testing or radiologic imaging like x-rays, CT scans, or MRI scans. Finally, I will briefly review your other medical and surgical history, as well as any medications you are currently taking.

What is the standard ENT physical exam?

Obviously, any good ENT will look in your ears, nose and mouth, and feel around your neck. I do that for every patient, not just sinus patients. For people with sinus complaints, I will spend a little extra time pressing over the sinuses in the forehead and the cheeks and taking a close look into the front of the nose.

What is nasal endoscopy?

Nasal endoscopy is a specialized diagnostic test that ENT doctors can perform. It involves placing a thin metal scope inside the nose to see to the back of the nasal cavity and also higher up inside the nose where the sinuses drain. The nasal endoscope looks like a thin metal straw and when it goes in the nose, it does feel a little unusual and uncomfortable but it's typically not painful. It does sometimes make people sneeze, so give me a little warning so I can duck out of the way! If you sneeze on me anyway, I won't be offended- it will certainly not be the first time or the last time that one of my patients sneezes on me.

The nasal endoscope is not able to see all the way inside your sinuses (unless you've had a FESS in the past), but I am able to see the areas of the nose where the sinuses are draining and can inspect these areas for signs of inflammation or infection. These signs include swelling, redness, polyps, or green/yellow drainage.

For billing purposes, nasal endoscopy is considered a diagnostic procedure, and sometimes patients are confused when they see it on their bills later. It sometimes shows up on your bill as a "surgical procedure." Depending on your insurance, the cost of the nasal endoscopy may or may not be included with your office visit. We'll let you know ahead of time if it will cost extra and how much your out of pocket costs will be. Unfortunately, there's really no way for me to adequately assess your sinuses without performing nasal endoscopy.

What is a CT scan and who should get one?

A CT scan is similar to an x-ray but provides

better detail and more information. The CT allows me to see inside of your sinuses and to look for signs of chronic inflammation or trapped mucus. I'm also able to see the dimensions and layout of your actual sinus openings. Any patient with a history of chronic sinusitis or recurrent acute sinusitis who wants to consider a sinus procedure should have a CT scan of the sinuses. People who get occasional sinus infections do not need a CT scan.

Do I need to do anything to prepare for a CT scan and is there any downtime afterward?

You do not need to do anything to prepare for a sinus CT scan. Again, it's just like an x-ray so there's no recovery period or any discomfort while you are being scanned. You may have had intravenous contrast if you've ever had a CT scan of another part of the body, but this is not needed for sinus CT scans. It is normally used in CT scans of the chest and abdomen, as well as some other parts of the body.

Does the CT scan need to be done at a hospital or imaging center?

Not if your doctor has an in-office CT scanner. I have had one of these machines in my main office in Kyle, Texas since March 2016. It has made life much easier for me and my sinus patients. Having a CT scanner in the office is very convenient for everyone. As a patient, you only need one appointment instead of three.

If I did not have a CT scanner, you would need to see me as a new patient, then go to a hospital or radiology center another day to have the CT scan, and then come back a third day to see me for another appointment to review the scan.

Another nice thing about office CT scanners is they usually expose you to much less x-ray radiation versus a conventional CT machine. The CT scanner I use in my office has less than 10% the amount of radiation versus a conventional CT scanner that hospitals or imaging centers use. The amount of x-rays you receive in my scanner is about the same as you would get lying on the beach every day for a week-long vacation, or flying in an airplane from Los Angeles to New York.

What happens after the full history, physical exam, nasal endoscopy and CT scan?

At this point, I will review all of the results with you and together we will decide the plan for treatment of your sinus problems. For most patients with chronic sinusitis or recurrent acute sinusitis, I recommend balloon sinuplasty, usually with reduction of the turbinates included.

If you and I decide that another procedure or a medical treatment is the best option, I will recommend that instead. I think it is very important to take your preferences into account, and I do my best to ensure that you leave your appointment with all your questions answered and feeling confident about the plan of treatment.

If I decide to proceed with balloon sinuplasty, what happens next?

My office staff will contact your insurance company for approval of the procedure. Some insurance companies will want to see records of your visit and will take one to two weeks to approve the procedure. In my experience, insurance companies in Texas are usually pretty good about approving the balloon sinuplasty procedure but some out-of-state insurance companies do not cover it. Once we hear from your insurance, we will call you to schedule your procedure and to let you know if there are any out-of-pocket costs for you.

What are the preparations I need to do prior to an office balloon sinuplasty?

I will prescribe you a pain medication called Norco, that you will take about one hour before coming for your procedure. This prescription is required by federal law to be a paper prescription that you take to the pharmacy, and you can pick it up from the office anytime up until the day before your procedure. Norco is a prescription pain medicine that contains hydrocodone and tylenol. If you are allergic to this medication, we can discuss another option. You will need to have someone drive you to and from your appointment for the balloon sinuplasty procedure.

Now, you know all about what will happen if you decide to make an appointment to see me for your sinus problems. If you decide to have the balloon sinuplasty, the next chapter will show you what will happen next.

7 WHAT HAPPENS ON THE DAY OF MY BALLOON SINUPLASTY PROCEDURE?

So, the big day has arrived! I hope you're not feeling nervous, but if you are, I've got ways of helping with that too. I also hope that you're excited about taking action to start feeling better and get lasting relief from your chronic sinusitis. This chapter will discuss what happens during your balloon sinuplasty procedure in my office.

What should I do the day of the procedure before coming into the office?

First of all, take a deep breath and try to relax. I've done a lot of these procedures by this point in my career, and they are not that big a deal. So, if you tend to get anxious, do your best to relax (easier said than done, I know…).

One hour before coming in to your appointment,

you should take your pain medication that I prescribed. It is okay for you to eat and drink as usual the day of the procedure. There's no need for you to fast ahead of time like you would if you were having surgery. Finally, you must have someone available to drive you to and from the procedure. You may already be sleepy before the procedure from taking the pain medication, and you will definitely be sleepy and in no condition to drive safely after the procedure.

What happens when you arrive at the office before Dr. Evans sees you?

My nurse will bring you back to the procedure room in the office. At this point, she will go over the procedure with you and you will sign a consent form which gives me permission to do the balloon sinuplasty, as well as anything else, such as turbinate reduction. She will then spray Afrin, which is a decongestant spray, into your nose as well as tetracaine, which is a numbing medication. These are the exact same nasal sprays we used at your first visit before I examined your nose with the nasal endoscope.

Finally, she will give you an injection into your upper arm of a medication called Versed, which is a light sedative. This medication will make you sleepy and relaxed during the procedure and will relieve any nerves or anxiety you might be feeling. Typically, about one third of my patients actually fall asleep during the procedure and two thirds are awake but very relaxed.

Is it possible to have the procedure without having any sedative?

For my first 20 or so balloon sinuplasties in the office, I offered patients the choice of having sedation versus no sedation. While most of the patients who chose not to have sedation did fine, there were several people who were clearly uncomfortable and this made the procedure significantly more difficult for me and for them. Since then, I have required everyone to take pain medication one hour before coming in and to have the Versed injection prior to the procedure. With this protocol, the procedures go much more smoothly and there is almost no significant discomfort during the procedure.

If you really really don't want sedation, I will consider this option for you, but I strongly encourage you to have it because it really does make the procedure go much easier.

Does Dr. Evans explain what will happen?

Yes. After my nurse gets you checked in, I will come in and see you and I will walk you through everything that will happen during your procedure and while you are in the office. I will explain the process of numbing the inside of your nose (the Evans protocol) and will also explain everything that you should expect to happen during the procedure and afterwards for the rest of the day. All your questions and concerns will get answered before I do anything to your nose.

Are family members or friends allowed to stay for the procedure?

Yes, if they want. Some family members and friends like to stay and watch. Others prefer to stay in the waiting room and a third group will leave and go get a snack and come back after the procedure. Whatever they want to do is fine with me. This is another benefit of an office procedure versus going to the operating room, because friends and family are never allowed in the OR.

What is the Evans protocol?

The Evans protocol is the method I've developed for keeping you as comfortable as possible during the balloon sinuplasty procedure in my office. I have developed this protocol through my experience and a bit of trial and error over the years. We already discussed the first part of the Evans protocol- the medications that help to keep you relaxed and comfortable. These are the Norco you take an hour before coming into the office and the Versed injection you get after your arrival.

There are then three steps for numbing the inside of your nose. The first step is the Afrin and tetracaine sprays that my nurse puts in your nose before I even see you. The second and third steps of the protocol are performed by me while using the nasal endoscope to see into your nose.

For the second step, I squirt a concentrated lidocaine gel over the area of the sinus openings and also lower in the nose over the septum and the turbinates. Lidocaine is a common medication that provides local anesthesia. The lidocaine gel is fairly thick, so it tends to stay where it is placed and doesn't immediately drip into the throat like a thinner liquid will. The gel sits inside your nose for about five minutes and actually works extremely well on its own.

However, just to be sure you will feel as little as possible inside your nose, I do perform a third step in the numbing protocol. The third step consists of several small injections of lidocaine around the sinus openings and into the turbinates if you are also having your turbinates shrunken. During these injections, no one feels the needle stick because the lining in the nose is already quite numb by this point. In over 150 of these balloon sinuplasty procedures in my office, I have never seen anyone jolt or really show any sign of discomfort at all during any needle injection I've done inside the nose.

Again, to review, the Evans protocol consists of 2 medications you get before the procedure and 3 steps of numbing the inside of your nose. I've been able to fine tune this process and have used it more than 150 patients with excellent results.

After I am fully relaxed and numbed inside my nose, how does the procedure typically go?

The way the procedure is done is I first look inside your nose with the nasal endoscope. The balloon device has a lighted guide wire that I'm able to gently thread through the sinus opening into the sinus. The openings for the frontal sinus and maxillary sinus are near each other in a part of the nose called the middle meatus. The opening for the sphenoid sinus is in the very back of the nasal cavity. For each sinus opening, I probe carefully with the guidewire until it falls into the sinus.

Once I have advanced the wire into the frontal or maxillary sinus, I can see the light on the end of the wire through the skin and know that I'm inside of the sinus. We keep the room dark during the procedure so I can see the guidewire light through the skin of the cheek or the forehead. With the sphenoid sinus, I can see or feel the sinus opening since it is a straight shot to the back of the nose.

Once I confirm that the wire is through the sinus opening, I advance the balloon over the wire through the sinus opening. Once it's sitting in the correct spot, my assistant will inflate the balloon with pressurized water, up to a pressure of 12 atmospheres. When this happens, you will feel some brief pressure and discomfort and hear some snap, crackle, and pop sounds as the sinus opening is permanently widened. The inflation lasts 5 seconds or so for each sinus that is stretched open during the procedure.

The balloon and guidewire are then pulled out and I move on to the next sinus opening. I can dilate up to 6 sinuses during any one procedure (the 2 maxillary, frontal, and sphenoid sinuses on each side). No splints or gauze packing are left inside the nose after the balloon sinuplasty.

Tell me about turbinate reduction.

As we said before, the turbinates are structures in the floor of your nose that are commonly swollen in people with sinus and allergy problems and take up a lot of space where air should be moving. In the majority of my balloon sinuplasty procedures, I also recommend to shrink the turbinates to help you breathe better. I have a probe that I can place inside the soft tissue of the turbinates, and it delivers an electric current that basically cooks the inside of each turbinate. Over the next several weeks, this "cooked" area will scar/contract and the turbinates will shrink down. This helps people to breathe better and is a very simple and easy thing to do, so I commonly perform it at the same time as balloon sinuplasty.

What happens at the end of my procedure before leaving the office?

After the procedure, I will place some gauze soaked in Afrin inside your nose for a few minutes. This helps to stop any minor bleeding. This gauze is removed and then I will fasten a folded gauze pad underneath your nose to catch any bleeding or oozing that comes out on the way home.

My staff will help you out of the office to the car that you're going to ride home in. Some patients are pretty sleepy so we do have a wheelchair available if necessary. You will receive a bag containing instructions, some extra gauze and a sample of a sinus rinse that you will start using the next day. We also give all the instructions to your spouse, relative, or friend who is driving you home because you may be drowsy and have a difficult time remembering everything the next day.

What happens the rest of the day after leaving the office?

Usually you will ride home and then take a nap for a few hours. Your throat will probably be numb for 2-3 hours after the procedure because some of the lidocaine gel always manages to drip into your throat. While your throat is numb, it will feel swollen and swallowing may be difficult until the numbing wears off. I recommend you do not try to eat or drink anything until your throat returns to normal. It is very easy to swallow the wrong way and choke yourself by accident. You will probably be sore and have moderate pain levels for one to two days, for which you can take the Norco I prescribed as needed.

Are there any warning signs of a serious complication to look for?

The main thing you should look out for is serious bleeding. A little minor bleeding and oozing is expected after balloon sinuplasty (with or without turbinate reduction), but if the gauze under your nose becomes saturated with blood in five minutes or less, I would be concerned about that. Please call me if this occurs or if there are any other unusual concerns. Fortunately, I have never seen severe bleeding like that happen in over 150 of these procedures.

The only time I have seen a problematic nosebleed after balloon sinuplasty was in one patient who took Warfarin (a blood-thinning medication). Although he had stopped this medication for a few days around the time of his procedure at my instruction, he did have a bad nosebleed that required nasal packing after he restarted his Warfarin 5 days after the procedure. That being said, I have had a number of other patients who restarted blood thinners after balloon sinuplasty with no problems at all.

Other concerning signs after balloon sinuplasty would be swelling or bruising around your eye, any change in your vision, or if you're having any dripping of clear fluid from your nose that tastes salty. These are signs of an injury to the eye socket or a leak of cerebrospinal fluid. Both of these potential complications are extremely rare, and I have thankfully never seen either of them in my practice.

How would this day be different if my balloon sinuplasty was done in the operating room instead?

Well, the procedure itself is done in exactly the same way in the operating room as I do it in the office. Since you are asleep under anesthesia, I obviously don't need to spend 20-30 minutes completing the Evans numbing protocol that I do in the office. You definitely will not feel anything during the procedure while you are under general anesthesia.

Other than that, there are a number of other differences. The first is that anything done in the operating room will take MUCH longer for you than in the office. Normally, you will be in my office for only about 1 hour total for a balloon sinuplasty procedure. In the operating room, you should usually plan to be there most of the day. You will usually be instructed to arrive at least 2 hours before your scheduled start time, and then you will be in the recovery room for a few hours after the procedure to allow you to wake up sufficiently from the anesthesia. There are frequently delays due to emergency procedures or the surgeon before me running late, so your procedure could easily start an hour or more later than scheduled.

The other major difference is that you have the additional risks of general anesthesia, and also the common side effects of anesthesia, such as nausea and vomiting afterward that can last for a day or more. These side effects rarely occur and are much less severe with the light sedation I use in the office.

So now you know the nitty gritty details of how the balloon sinuplasty procedure works in my office. We will now move on to what happens in the days, weeks, and months after having the procedure.

8 WHAT HAPPENS AFTER MY BALLOON SINUPLASTY PROCEDURE?

You've had your balloon sinuplasty procedure. Now what?

Keep reading to find out! This chapter will talk about the typical things that happen during the time you are recovering after the procedure. It is important to note that these are the average things that happen. Most patients will be similar to what I describe in this chapter, but some have an easier time and some have a harder time.

What should I start doing the morning after my procedure?

Starting the morning after your balloon sinuplasty procedure, I want you to start rinsing your nose with saline at least twice a day. This can be done with a sinus rinse kit or with a Neti Pot. There are many different brands of sinus rinse that all should work about the same- I typically recommend NeilMed, which is easy to find at drug stores and grocery stores. We'll give you a sample NeilMed rinse bottle the day of your procedure to take home.

Make sure to buy distilled water to mix in your sinus rinse instead of using tap water. There have been rare reports of life-threatening infections caused by an amoeba called Naegleria that is rarely found in tap water. This infection is extremely rare, but it is not something you want to take a chance on.

Also, on the day after your procedure, you can start blowing your nose very gently but avoid any strong nose blowing because this can cause bleeding. I also prefer you to avoid any straining or strenuous exercise for at least three days after the procedure because this can also cause bleeding.

What is the first week like after my procedure?

Usually you will have some moderate pain and soreness for one to two days after the procedure. Then, for the next five to seven days, you typically just feel stuffy, congested and have some pressure in their sinus areas. There may be increased green or yellow drainage. You may feel feel like you are getting a sinus infection, and the symptoms following balloon sinuplasty are actually very similar to sinusitis in many patients. You also may notice some crusting inside your nose- this is a combination of dried blood and mucus and usually forms on the turbinates while they are healing. There is rarely any significant crusting in or around the sinuses from the balloon procedure.

What happens during the second week after my procedure?

Usually after about one week, the pressure and congestion in your nose and face start improving a lot. At this time, it is okay for you to start using Flonase or any other of your usual allergy medications again. You will probably still notice some crusting in your nose that you can gently blow out or rinse out with saline. Please continue using your sinus rinses at least twice a day- this is very important to allow for proper healing and good long-term results.

When is my first office appointment after the procedure and what happens during it?

The first post-procedure appointment is usually about two weeks after you had your balloon sinuplasty. At this time, I will check in with you and see how you are feeling. If necessary, I can pull crusts out of your nose, which will help you to feel better right away. I will also perform a nasal endoscopy and look around the areas of the sinus openings and where any work was done. Usually at this stage of healing, I will see some minor swelling from the procedure but things are starting to look much better and more open than before the balloon sinuplasty.

What happens over the next month after my first office visit?

You will gradually start to feel better and better. I strongly urge you to continue to flush your nose with saline at least twice a day during this time. Some patients will notice an increase in drainage from their nose, and the reason for this is your sinuses are now able to drain properly! It can take a few weeks up to a few months for your sinuses to fully clear themselves out and dry up. The crusting in your nose will gradually go away over this period of time and you will really start to feel the benefit of the procedure and begin feeling much better.

What happens at the second post-procedure visit?

At your second visit back with me, about 6 weeks after the procedure, I will again check in with you and see how you're doing. I will perform nasal endoscopy and take one more look at the sinuses and the turbinates. Usually by this time, everything is completely healed and there's no further crusting. During your appointment, I will have you fill out another Sino-Nasal Outcome Test survey (SNOT-20) and we can compare the survey from today to the survey you completed before your balloon sinuplasty and normally we'll see a great improvement on this. About 85% of my patients have more than a 20% reduction in their symptom score, and about 65% of my patients have a greater than 50% reduction in their sinus symptoms.

At this time, it is also okay for you to stop rinsing your nose every day. I have found that many patients start to enjoy their sinus rinses and will continue doing them for the long run. But if you think that rinsing your nose is like being waterboarded, you can stop!

What is the long term follow up after my second post-procedure appointment?

After the second appointment, my hope is that you will continue to enjoy the benefits of your procedure for the foreseeable future. There are a few long-term medical research studies which show a lasting improvement for over 5 years after having balloon sinuplasty. Since the procedure has only been around for 10 years or so, we don't have longer-term data than that, but I suspect that a large number of patients will get permanent improvement in their sinusitis from balloon sinuplasty.

After you complete the healing process, you should be breathing better, have less sinus pressure and less sinus infections. If you did not get better from the procedure, we will re-evaluate and look for other options. Normally, I will have you follow up with me 3 to 4 months later to keep an eye on you and make sure we are controlling your allergies properly and look out for any problems before they become serious.

Does anyone ever need balloon sinuplasty a second or third time?

Out of the 150+ balloon sinuplasty procedures I've performed, I've only repeated the procedure on one patient. Normally, I would only consider repeating balloon sinuplasty if it worked for some period of time but then the patient had a recurrence of their chronic sinusitis.

That's exactly what happened with the one patient I mentioned. He had a balloon sinuplasty in 2013 and felt great for about two years. Unfortunately, then he started feeling worse again and his CT scan confirmed that his chronic sinusitis had recurred. Since he had his second balloon sinuplasty in late 2016, he has been feeling well.

That's really the only situation for which I would consider repeating the procedure. If someone has balloon sinuplasty and it doesn't help them at all, it doesn't make sense to try it again in my opinion. Fortunately, with proper selection of patients (i.e. people who really have chronic sinusitis or recurrent acute sinusitis, not something else), balloon sinuplasty works very well for 80-90% of patients.

Now you are more of an expert on sinus disorders and procedures than almost anyone, including most non-ENT doctors. But we left out one very important topic: the effects of balloon sinuplasty on your bank account! As we wrap up this book, we'll talk for a bit about the finances of balloon sinuplasty.

9 HOW MUCH DOES BALLOON SINUPLASTY COST?

Can I use my health insurance to help pay for balloon sinuplasty?

Yes, most people do use their health insurance for this procedure. In Texas, almost all of the insurance companies cover balloon sinuplasty. Some insurance companies make us jump through a lot of hoops to get these procedures approved, but almost all of them will cover it in the end. I have run into some out-of-state insurance plans that do not cover the procedure.

If you and I decide that balloon sinuplasty is the right treatment for you, my office staff will contact your insurance for approval. This process is known as pre-authorization. Every insurance company has a different process. Some of them will approve the procedure with no hassle. Others require that we send records of your office visit and CT scan and will take

1-2 weeks reviewing them to ensure that you meet their criteria for having the procedure.

What are Dr. Evans's costs for the procedure?

It does cost me a pretty good amount of money to do these procedures. I think it is helpful for you to understand why the price tag for balloon sinuplasty is fairly high. Unfortunately, the amount paid you might see on your insurance statements does not all go into my pocket.

The amount I get paid for each balloon sinuplasty procedure is different and depends on how many sinuses get dilated and also how much each different insurance plan pays. Whatever amount I get paid that is greater than the cost of the balloon device and the other necessary medications and equipment is my profit. Each balloon device that I use is only used one time for your procedure and then is thrown away. The cost for me of each balloon device, the medications and other necessary equipment for your procedure is several thousand dollars.

How much are my out-of-pocket costs for balloon sinuplasty?

The answer to this question totally depends on your insurance. Some patients will pay nothing out of pocket for balloon sinuplasty. Other patients will only pay their typical specialist's office copay (usually in the $20-$60 range) and the cost of the procedure is covered within that payment. And finally some patients may be required by their insurance plan to pay more because the cost of the procedure goes toward their annual deductible. This amount could be several hundred or even potentially a few thousand dollars, depending on the insurance stipulations.

Unfortunately there is no easy way to tell ahead of your first visit with me how much the procedure will cost. Once you have been evaluated by me and we have settled on the specific plan for the procedure (i.e. how many sinuses will be dilated, whether the turbinates will be reduced in size, etc), we will be able to contact your insurance company for an accurate estimate of your costs.

Is balloon sinuplasty less expensive in the operating room?

Generally, no. In the operating room, you and your insurance not only have to pay a fee for my services, there's also a fee to the surgical facility and then another fee to the anesthesiologist. Usually the cost for you will be either the same as in the office or more expensive. It is very unlikely to be less expensive. The cost that your insurance company pays is usually quite a bit more in a hospital or surgery center than in the office.

Will I know ahead of time how much the procedure will cost?

Yes. My office staff will contact your insurance company to find out this information once you have decided you want to proceed with having balloon sinuplasty (or any other procedure or surgery, for that matter). Once we know this information, my staff will call you to schedule the procedure and will let you know your out-of-pocket costs at that time.

Does Dr. Evans offer payment plans?

Yes. We offer Care Credit, which allows some patients to have no interest loans for procedures, as well as other financing options. Care Credit has its own qualification process to determine if you are eligible for their credit line. For patients who do not qualify for Care Credit, we are sometimes able to offer customized payment plans.

What is the balloon sinuplasty procedure really worth to me?

This is a question you have to ask yourself. What is permanent improvement in your sinus problems worth to you? If you are a young or a middle aged person, you most likely have decades of life ahead of you. What is it worth to you to feel healthy during that time? It's easy to get caught up worrying about spending a few hundred dollars or even a few thousand dollars but sometimes it may be worth it to spend that money. My office staff and I are very willing to work with you to help with payment plans or other ways to make these procedures affordable for you if you really need them.

10 CONCLUSION

Let's wrap this book up, and recap what we learned! I'll keep it very short, like the rest of this book. I want you to take action to start feeling better, not sit around for hours reading a thick textbook!

In the early chapters, we learned about what sinusitis is and what it isn't. We learned about the major symptoms of sinusitis, including pressure in the face, stuffy nose, thick drainage from the nose, and loss of smell. We learned about medications used for sinusitis as well as allergy testing and treatment of specific allergies. I described to you the history of sinus surgery and its evolution from more invasive and crude forms into the minimally invasive procedures we see today. I then discussed my philosophy of treating chronic sinusitis and why I think that balloon sinuplasty is the right choice to try first for the majority of patients.

Finally, we focused on what your experience

would be in my practice if you decided to come in for an appointment and then proceeded to have balloon sinuplasty.

Now it is up to you. Just because you have read this book, you don't necessarily have a sinus problem or need a sinus procedure. But you should have a pretty good idea of whether you need to see an ENT doctor for further evaluation of your sinus health.

So, what is the next step for you? If you are interested in seeing me, you can contact me via my website at TexanENT.com or the phone number to reach my office is 512-550-0321. For a limited time, I am offering free screening appointments for patients who believe they have chronic sinusitis. Please call today to set up your appointment.

11 RESOURCES

Here are some resources for you to learn more about me as well as other topics related to sinusitis and sinus surgery.

More Information about Dr. Seth Evans:

My practice's website: www.texanent.com

My professional blog: drsethevans.com

My professional Facebook page: facebook.com/drsethevans

PubMed.com - Online database created by the National Institutes of Health which contains millions of medical journal articles for you to search.

SinusVideos.com - This website shows short vide of a variety of different sinus surgeries, including balloon sinuplasty. Please note that some of the balloon sinuplasty videos show a different device with a rigid metal probe- this is not the device I use in my balloon procedures.

BalloonSinuplasty.com - This is a useful website created by Acclarent, the company that developed the balloon device that I use in my procedures.

ABOUT THE AUTHOR

Dr. Seth Evans has extensive experience in all areas of otolaryngology- head and neck surgery and sees patients of all ages. He has a particular interest in sinus disorders and minimally invasive surgery.

Dr. Evans is a born and raised Virginian who realized that he was a Texan at heart after visiting his younger sister who lived in the Austin area several years ago. After completing his otolaryngology residency in 2010, Dr. Evans some time traveling to Australia, New Zealand, Peru, and many parts of Europe. He moved to Central Texas in late 2011 and started his practice at Texan ENT Specialists full time in January 2012.

In his spare time, he enjoys tormenting his friends and family in the north with weather reports of the Texas "winter," attending live music shows, trying to break 80 on the golf course, stuffing himself with beef brisket, and spending time with his wife and family.

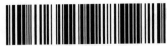

Made in the USA
San Bernardino, CA
23 May 2018